Infection Control in Hea............ ....
Guidebook

By Daniel Farb, M.D., Bruce Gordon

By the same authors…

<u>Bioterrorism Certificate Program</u> received five stars from ForewordReviews.com: "Timely and thorough."

<u>OSHA Bloodborne Pathogens</u> received five stars from ForewordReviews.com: "Required reading for all who work in a healthcare setting."

<u>Total Quality in Provider Practices</u> received five stars from ForewordReviews.com: "Excellent tool to assist any health care organization."

Please send any correspondence regarding permissions to:
UniversityOfHealthCare
419 N. Larchmont Blvd., #323
Los Angeles, CA 90004

Infection Control in Healthcare Facilities Guidebook

ISBN 13: 9781594912917
ISBN 10: 1594912912

Library of Congress Catalog Number: 2006902058

UniversityOfHealthCare/ UniversityOfBusiness website:
www.uohc.com

Contents

Introduction

This book is a text-only version of our acclaimed CD on Infection Control in Healthcare Facilities. We have made it for those who prefer books.

The purpose of this guidebook is to help the user understand and implement important standards for an infection control program. It is perfect for clinical and administrative staff.

We recommend that, if you have training needs or need to document your mastery of this material, you obtain the CD also.

About the Authors

M. Daniel Farb, CEO of UniversityOfHealthCare and UniversityOfBusiness, is a leader in the field of interactive management and healthcare e-learning. He received a BA in English Literature from Yale (where he set an academic record and studied with writers like Robert Penn Warren), an M.D. from Boston University, a degree in Executive Management from the Anderson School of Business at UCLA, and is currently working on a degree at UCLA in International Trade. He is a practicing ophthalmologist. He also has received two patents in ophthalmology and is working on others, has worked with the World Health Organization in Geneva and the National Institutes of Health in Washington, D.C. He has written scientific and popular articles, and has worked as a newspaper reporter. He helped Dr. Robbins edit one of the editions of Robbins' "Pathology" textbook for readability. He wrote an article on humor for the Massachusetts Review. He has experience in theater and television, including acting, directing, and stage-managing. He has programmed his own patient records database. He has written and edited hundreds of e-learning courses.

Dr. Farb is a member of the American Academy of Ophthalmology, the Union of American Physicians and Dentists, the AOJS, the American Association of Physicians and Surgeons, the ASTD (American Society for Training and Development), the E-Learning Forum, the Southern California Biomedical Council, the PDA (Parenteral Drug Association), and the Medical Marketing Association.

BRUCE GORDON is the Creative Director for UniversityOfHealthCare, LLC, and plays an important role in writing the more creative projects, especially those with stories.

After receiving a BA in Economics from UCLA, he began a freelance writing career that included technical writing (such as a manual for Princess Cruise Lines), stand-up comedy routines for nationally known comedians, and screenplay writing. He has done production support work with famous Hollywood personalities on such well-known productions as Aaron Spelling's "Dynasty" and "Love Boat" TV shows.

An audio-visual software specialist, he is a versatile artist, with published works in a variety of media, including music, motion graphics, and digital video short film.

Infection Control in Healthcare Facilities

Objectives

Upon the completion of this course, you will be able to...
1. List JCAHO standards and requirements for infection control
2. Illustrate JCAHO's primary focus areas of surveillance, prevention, and control
3. Describe personnel issues in infection control
4. Demonstrate detailed prevention procedures
5. Summarize the hierarchy of decontamination
6. Describe emergency management concerns

Surveillance, Prevention, and Control of Infection

It is a disturbing and ironic fact that too many people enter a hospital or other healthcare setting for one reason, and end up sick for other non-related reasons. These buildings are full of disease-causing agents, even though they are supposed to be where people come to get well, not ill. Although the potential risks for this have always existed, it seems that the dangers have increased. Some of the reasons for this are:
* More advanced and invasive surgical techniques and treatment regimens
* An increase in severity of patient illness
* A shortage of nurses in the field

Around 90,000 deaths occur every year from these healthcare-associated infections (otherwise known as HAIs). Based on the fact that about two million people are admitted to acute care hospitals, this puts the percentage of deaths somewhere near 5%. Not only do the Centers for Disease Control and Prevention (CDC) and other authorities feel that this is too many, they also think that one-third of them are preventable.

The CDC also estimates that, in addition to the human costs, the financial impact of treating this excess of infections reaches close to $5 billion.

Here are examples of the major reasons for the high numbers afflicted in a healthcare setting. In a long-term care facility, highly susceptible elderly patients are further vulnerable because of:
* Illnesses increasing in severity
* Transfer from hospitals at a rapid rate
* Staff turnover that is very high
* The lack of available private rooms
* Ventilation system inadequacies
* Other factors

Besides long-term care facilities, other healthcare settings are complicated by infections. Some of these are:
* Clinics
* Surgery centers
* Dialysis centers
* Home care

Some infectious diseases have never been susceptible to or have become resistant to known drugs. These diseases account for 70% of HAIs. Some of the major ones are:
* Methicillin Resistant Staphylococcus Aureus (MRSA)
* Vancomycin Resistant Enterocolitis (VRE)
* Hepatitis
* Tuberculosis (TB)
* HIV

Other HAIs are caused by the presence of airborne or waterborne microbes, which fall under a category called environmental failures. Every year, two to three thousand deaths occur from these types.

Because the best way to deal with HAIs is from the standpoint of prevention, it should be a priority for any organization that is committed to safety initiatives. Each healthcare organization should institute an infection control (IC) program to evaluate and design a systematic approach to mitigate HAI-related problems.

Research has identified some of the major direct causes of HAIs, as well as ways in which to control them. This is also the case for many of the behaviors and situations that result in high risk. Even with the fact that underlying diseases are impossible to avoid, many strides have been made in controlling their spread.

The Joint Commission on Accreditation of Healthcare Organizations (JCAHO) has established a goal of reducing the risk of acquisition and transmission of HAIs via the use of effective IC programs. JCAHO has made specific determinations about how an effective infection prevention and control program should be structured and applied. Required are:
* An integrated, responsive process
* The collaboration by numerous programs, services, and settings throughout the hospital (or other healthcare setting)
* The development, implementation, and evaluation of the IC program by all in the organization.

The risks that the hospital faces in respect to infectious disease acquisition and transmission will determine the IC program's design and scope.

What should hospitals do to prevent HAIs?
* The organization's safety and performance improvement programs need to include infection control as one of their prime directives.
* The organization needs to locate its risks for infectious agent acquisition and transmission and perform this assessment on an ongoing basis.
* The organization needs to employ an approach based upon epidemiology by focusing on surveillance, data collection, and trend identification.
* The organization needs to institute infection prevention and control processes and follow up on them constantly.
* The organization needs to educate and collaborate with leaders throughout the organization about participating in the IC program design and implementation.
* The organization needs to be aware that infection control is a community wide effort, and it needs to blend its efforts with those of other healthcare and community leaders.
* The organization needs to make plans for responding to a possible situation in which its resources become overwhelmed by a catastrophic number of infections. This allows the hospital or other healthcare facility to remain a practical resource in the community.

It is imperative that hospital leaders become and stay directly involved in the IC program. This is the only way in which it can be properly resourced and the only way the proper scope can be determined.

JCAHO has established primary focus areas (PFAs) for healthcare organization's IC programs. These include:
* Surveillance/identification
* Prevention
* Control

These PFAs are designed to be applied in a system-wide, integrated process that covers all programs, services, and settings. They also have to be adhered to by everyone in the hospital, including:
* Patients
* Employees
* Physicians
* Other licensed independent practitioners
* Contract service workers
* Volunteers
* Students
* Visitors

Detecting changes in infection trends is the main purpose of the surveillance or identification area primary focus area. To locate trouble or negative trends, surveillance data must be employed. Whether to gain positive feedback or guidance for improving performance, the trended data is important to the needs of various leadership and line staff members.

Besides identifying risks and problems, an organization has to be active in preventing the occurrence of infections. There are a multitude of prevention measures and techniques. Briefly, some of them include:
* Giving vaccine to staff or patients who are at risk for hepatitis B. These could include hemodialysis patients, those with hemophilia, and substance abusers.
* Making sure that standard precautions are employed
* Screening for and administering pneumococcal and influenza vaccines for the appropriate patients and employees. This includes childhood vaccines, too.

To combat the possibility of exposure to chickenpox for workers in pediatric settings and long-term care facilities, Varicella screening and vaccination are important.
* Administration of a Kwell bath to indigent patients, as well as those with poor self-care.
* Following the The Centers for Disease Control and Prevention (CDC) guidelines on immunizing health care workers (HCWs), other adults, and children.
* Cleaning, disinfecting, and sterilizing equipment properly. Appropriate sanitation of the environment is included in this area.

Reporting of all reportable infections or diseases must be executed by the organization:
* Externally, as mandated by regulation and law
* Internally, incorporating the information into the organization's surveillance and performance improvement procedures, as well as its sentinel event process (as pertinent).

Along with internal discussions on surveillance reports, the organization really should strive to stay aware of infectious-disease syndromes that may be occurring in the community (by establishing and maintaining a close liaison with local public health agencies).

In regards to the data for measuring the effectiveness of actions and outcomes, the organization should take great lengths to:
* Collect it
* Analyze it
* Investigate it
* Share it with top management (and others, as appropriate)

The outcomes of this IC data will influence many other activities of the organization, including:

* The overall safety program
* Performance improvement (PI)
* Pharmacy and therapeutics (PT)
* Peer review
* Credentialing

Here are some specific examples of IC activities:
* Hand washing
* Using personal protective equipment
* Precaution and isolation procedures
* Cleaning procedures for disinfecting and/or sterilization
* Ongoing measurement of performance

JCAHO Standards and Requirements

The first set of IC standards fall under the heading of "The JCAHO Infection Control Program and Its Components."

Standard IC.1.10 - IC Program
(The Goal)
The risk of development of a health care-associated infection (HAI) needs to be minimized through an organization-wide infection control program.

It's important to achieve this goal because, throughout the hospital, there are always risks of HAIs. This means that it's imperative to include all pertinent settings and programs of the hospital in order to systematically locate risks and offer the proper response.

To achieve this goal, the following steps need to be taken:
1. An organization-wide IC program needs to be implemented.

2. Individuals and/or positions with the authority to take steps to prevent or control the acquisition and transmission of infectious agents should be identified.

3. All applicable organization components and functions need to be integrated into the IC program.

4. Systems need to be in place to communicate with all relevant persons about infection prevention and control issues, including their responsibilities in preventing the spread of infection within the hospital. This can include

* Licensed independent practitioners (LIPs)
* Staff
* Students and trainees
* Volunteers
* Visitors and patients, as pertinent

5. The hospital needs to have systems for reporting identified infections to the following entities:

* Appropriate hospital staff
* Federal, state, and local public health authorities in as mandated by law and regulation
* Accrediting bodies, per Sentinel Event Reporting and National Patient Safety Goals publications
* The referring or receiving organization in the case where a patient was transferred or referred and the presence of an infection wasn't known at the time of transfer of referral

6. Systems need to be in place for investigating outbreaks of infectious diseases.

7. Applicable policies and procedures need to be in place throughout the hospital.

8. The hospital needs to maintain a written IC plan that includes:

* An itemization of prioritized risks, along with their descriptions
* The IC program goals in a written statement

* A listing of the hospital's strategies to minimize, reduce, or eliminate the prioritized risks, along with itemized descriptions
* Information on how the organization will evaluate the strategies.

The written plan needs to be a succinct and useful document that:
* Identifies needs
* Itemizes strategies to meet those needs
* Sets objectives and goals
* Includes narratives, policies and procedures, protocols, and approved practices in the plan's format

Standard IC.2.10 - Identify Risks
(The Goal)
The infection control program needs to identify risks for the acquisition and transmission of infectious agents on an ongoing basis.

It's important to do this because a hospital's risks of infection will vary based on:
* The hospital's geographic location
* The community environment
* Services provided
* The characteristics and behaviors of the population served.
Risk assessment needs to be an ongoing process, since these risks will invariably change, and sometimes rapidly.

Achievement of this goal will require the following steps:
1. The hospital needs to identify risks for the transmission and acquisition of infectious agents throughout the hospital based on the following factors:
* The geographic location and community environment of the hospital, services provided, and the characteristics of the population served

* The results of the analysis of the hospital's infection prevention and control data
* The care, treatment, and services provided
2. At least annually and whenever significant changes occur in any of the factors just mentioned, the risk analysis needs to be formally reviewed.
3. Surveillance activities need to be employed to identify infection prevention and control risks pertaining to:
* Patients
* LIPs, staff, volunteers, students, and trainees
* Visitors, as appropriate

Standard IC.3.10 - Priorities and Goals
(The Goal)
The hospital needs to establish priorities (based on risks), and then set goals for preventing the development of health care-associated infections within the hospital.

This goal is important because, while a healthcare organization's resources are usually limited, the HAI risks within the hospital are numerous. To have an effective IC program, the hospital needs to have a thoughtful prioritization of the most important risks to be addressed.

The choice and design of strategies for infection prevention and control in a hospital need to be guided by the priorities and goals related to the identified risks, which also supply a framework for evaluating the strategies.

To be successful at this goal, the following steps need to be taken: Based on the risks identified, priorities have to be established and goals have to be developed in the plan for preventing the acquisition and transmission of potentially infectious agents.

A partial list of these goals includes:
* Limiting unprotected exposure to pathogens throughout the hospital
* Enhancing hand hygiene guidelines, clinical paths, care maps, or a combination of these
* Minimizing the risk of transmission of infections associated with the use of procedures, medical equipment, and medical devices

Standard IC.4.10 Strategies – Screening - Isolation
(The Goal)
Once the hospital has prioritized its goals, strategies need to be implemented to achieve the goals.

To be effective, it's necessary for the hospital to plan and implement interventions to address the IC issues that it finds important, and to base them on prioritized risks and associated surveillance data.

To accomplish this mandate, these steps should be executed:
Interventions need to be designed to incorporate relevant guidelines for infection prevention and control activities.
* An organization-wide hand hygiene program that complies with current CDC hand hygiene guidelines
* Methods to reduce the risks associated with procedures, medical equipment, and medical devices including the following:
  - Appropriate storage, cleaning, disinfection, sterilization, and/or disposal of supplies and equipment
  - Reuse of equipment designated by the manufacturer as disposable in a manner that is consistent with regulatory and professional standards
  - The appropriate use of personal protective equipment

* Implementation of applicable precautions as appropriate are based upon:
  - The potential for transmission
  - The mechanism of transmission
  - The care setting
  - The emergence and reemergence of pathogens in the community that could affect the hospital
* Screening must be available as needed for exposure and/or immunity to infectious diseases that LIPs, staff, students/trainees, and volunteers may come in contact within the course of their work.
* For LIPs, staff, students/trainees, and volunteers who are identified as potentially having an infectious disease or risk of infectious disease that may put the population they serve at risk, appropriate referrals need to be made as for:
  -- Assessment
  -- Potential testing
  -- Immunization
  -- Prophylaxis and treatment
  -- Counseling
* For patients, students/trainees, and volunteers who have been exposed to infectious disease(s) at the hospital and LIPs or staff who are occupationally exposed, appropriate referrals need to be made for:
  -- Assessment
  -- Potential testing
  -- Immunization
  -- Prophylaxis and treatment
  -- Counseling
* Reduction of risks associated with animals brought into the hospital

Standard IC.5.10 - Evaluation of Effectiveness
(The Goal)

The infection control program needs to evaluate the effectiveness of the infection control interventions. It also needs to redesign the infection control interventions, as necessary.

This is an important goal to achieve, since the evaluation of the effectiveness of interventions helps to identify which activities of the IC program are effective and which activities need to be changed to improve outcomes. This goal can be attained by the following steps:
* The hospital needs to formally evaluate and annually revise the goals and program (or portions of the program). Additional evaluations and revisions need to be done whenever risks are significantly changed.
* The evaluation needs to address changes in the scope of the IC program that come from such areas as the introduction of:
  -- New services
  -- New sites of care
* The evaluation also needs to address changes in the results of the IC program risk analysis
* The evaluation further must address emerging and reemerging problems (such as highly infectious agents) in the health care community that potentially affect the hospital.
* The evaluation must finally address the following:
  -- The assessment of the success or failure of interventions for preventing and controlling infection.
  -- Responses to concerns raised by leadership and others within the hospital.
  -- The evolution of relevant infection prevention and control guidelines that are based on evidence. When this evidence is not available, expert consensus is used.

Standard IC.6.10 – Emergency Response
(The Goal)

As part of emergency management activities, the organization needs to prepare to respond to an influx, or the risk of an influx, of infectious patients.

This goal is very important because of the importance that healthcare organizations have as resources to help the community function continually. There is a definite threat to an organization's ability to deliver services when catastrophic problems, which are likely to require expanded or extended care capabilities over a prolonged period of time, occur in the community. This could render the organization ill prepared to respond to an epidemic or infections.

This makes it imperative that the organization plan how to:
* Prevent the introduction of the infection into the organization
* Quickly recognize that this type of infection has been introduced
* Contain the spread of the infection if it is introduced

What are some of the options of this planned response?
* The temporary halting of services and/or admissions
* Delaying transfer or discharge
* Limiting visitors within an organization
* Fully activating the organization's emergency management plan

Of course, the actual response will be based in addressing such issues as:
* The extent to which the community is affected by the spread of the infection
* The types of services offered
* The capabilities of the organization

Here's how this can be accomplished:

1. The organization needs to plan its response to an influx or risk of an influx of infectious patients.
2. The organization needs to have a plan for managing an ongoing influx of potentially infectious patients/residents/clients over an extended period of time.
3. The organization:
* Figures out how it will stay abreast of current information about the emergence of epidemics or new infections that may result in the organization activating its response
* Develops a plan to disseminate critical information to staff and other key practitioners
* Distinguishes which community resources can provide additional information. These can include local, state, and or federal public health systems.

The next set of IC standards fall under the heading of "Structure and Resources for the JCAHO Infection Control Program."

Standard IC.7.10 – Infection Control Program
(The Goal)
The infection control program has to be managed effectively.

The importance of this goal lies in the fact that the IC program requires management by an individual (or individuals) with knowledge that is appropriate to the risks identified by the hospital, as well as knowledge of:
* The analysis of infection risks
* Principles of infection prevention and control
* Data analysis

The person fulfilling this requirement may be employed by the hospital or the hospital may contract with him or her. The hospital's size, complexity, and needs will determine how many of these individuals are needed and on what to base their qualifications.

What does the hospital need to do to make this goal a reality?
1. The hospital needs to assign responsibility for managing IC program activities to one or more individuals whose number, competency, and skill mix are determined by the goals and objectives of the IC activities.
2. Qualifications of the individual(s) responsible for managing the IC program need to be determined by the risks entailed in the services provided, the hospital's patient population(s), and the complexity of the activities that will be carried out. Ongoing education, training, experience, and/or certification [such as that offered by the Certification Board for Infection Control (CBIC) in the prevention and control of infections] can help the individual meet the qualification requirements.
3. The individual or individuals coordinate all infection prevention and control within the hospital.
4. The individual or individuals facilitate ongoing monitoring of the effectiveness of prevention and/or control activities and interventions.

Standard IC.8.10 - Executive Support – IC Committee – Responsibilities

(The Goal)

Representatives from relevant components/functions within the hospital need to collaborate to implement the infection control program.

Why is this an important goal?
This is an important goal because any successful creation of an organization-wide IC program requires collaboration with all

relevant components/functions. This collaboration is so very critical to:
* The successful gathering and interpretation of data
* The design of interventions
* The effective implementation of interventions

Another mandate is that managers within the hospital who have the power to implement plans and make decisions about interventions related to infection prevention and control must participate in the IC program. A hospital might want to think about the option of establishing a formal committee consisting of leadership and other components, even though this isn't required as evidence of this collaboration.

This goal can be achieved by the following.
1. Ongoing collaboration between:
* The qualified personnel managing the IC program
* Hospital leaders including medical staff, LIPs
* Other direct and indirect patient care staff (including, when applicable, pharmacy, laboratory, administration, central supply/sterilization services, housekeeping, building maintenance/engineering, and food services)
2. Participation of these representatives needs to occur in:
* Development of strategies for each component's/function's role in the IC program
* Assessment of the adequacy of the human, information, physical, and financial resources allocated to support infection prevention and control activities
* Assessment of the overall failure or success of key processes for preventing and controlling infection
* The review and revision of the IC program as necessary to improve outcomes

Standard IC.9.10 - Adequate Resources and Structure

(The Goal)

Hospital leaders need to allocate adequate resources for the infection control program.

The reason that this goal is important is that, to effectively plan and successfully implement a program of this scope, adequate resources are needed.

This goal can be successfully implemented with the following steps:
1. On an ongoing basis (but no less frequently than annually), leaders need to review the effectiveness of the hospital's infection prevention and control activities and report their findings to the integrated patient safety program.
2. Adequate systems to access information must be provided to support infection prevention and control activities.
3. Adequate laboratory support needs to be provided to support infection prevention and control activities, when applicable.
4. Adequate equipment and supplies need to be provided to support infection prevention and control activities.

General Surveillance

Surveillance is the first primary focus area of a good IC program. It involves the gathering of infections-related data to:
* Evaluate an organization's infection risks by locating areas that need further investigation, such as areas where patients seem to be at higher or lower risk than before
* Locate any problems such as the emergence of new infections or outbreaks, such as Severe Acute Respiratory Syndrome (SARS) or influenza
* Hunt for cases of a specific disease

* Ascertain whether processes used to prevent and control infections are operating properly, as well as whether the systems need improvements or revisions
* Look into the success (or lack thereof) of any changes made to a system or process

What are some of the factors that cause an organization's IC risks to vary?
* Geographic location
* Community environment
* Services provided
* Population served, their characteristics, and behaviors

An illustration of this: A behavioral health care facility supplying residential, food pantry, and drop-in employment services may not have the same types of infection risks as an ambulatory surgery center.

Collecting data and assessing risks have to be ongoing activities, as part of a perpetual process, since infection risks change as time goes on. Since this has been shown to help prevent many healthcare- associated infections, this constant monitoring is more cost effective than resource intensive.

The determination of whether or not an IC program is really working as leadership needs it to can only be made with the quantitative information the organization gets from data collection and measurement activities.

Here are some details regarding the surveillance data that an organization collects and analyzes:
* It shows changes in infection trends
* It should be simple and practical.
* IC professionals use it to implement the IC program

* It needs to be quickly understood by all IC personnel, particularly in smaller organizations and non-acute settings where IC is added to their already voluminous duties.
* It needs to be focused on areas that impact patient safety and care outcomes the most, since resources are usually scarce.

An illustration of this is urinary tract infections. Since total surveillance of all such infections may not be possible, an effective monitoring strategy might involve:
* Only those with indwelling Foley catheters
* Only those with intermittent urinary catheters
* Limiting it to the time frame within which the infection would be considered organization associated

Targeted surveillance

Sometimes it's necessary to focus on particular patient procedures or populations. Here's an illustration involving a home care organization:

The monitoring of patients who receive enteral or parenteral feedings and who suffer a higher-than-expected incidence of diarrhea. This can uncover infection rate changes, as well as illuminate areas where improvement is needed.

Problem-oriented surveillance

Other times, the occurrence of specific infections in multiple patients at the same time needs to be measured. An example of this is when a group of patients are all afflicted with the same illness and data needs to be obtained to determine:
* Whether an ongoing problem exists
* What control measures can be used to bring the problem to resolution

As stated before, surveillance data collection will differ for organizations based on their patient populations and the services they provide. However, some common areas and groups to monitor have been identified, and should definitely be included in an organization's emergence management plans.

SARS is a main consideration, being the first severe and readily transmittable disease of this century, according to many public health officials. Some others are:
* Emerging pathogens such as West Nile Virus or Hepatitis C
* Bioterrorism agents (chemicals, and biologics such as smallpox)
* Multidrug-resistant tuberculosis
* Other respiratory viruses (such as RSV, para-influenza)
* Anthrax
* Multiple drug-resistant organisms, such as methicillin-resistant Staphylococcus aureus (MRSA) infections or vancomycin-resistant enterococci (VRE) (especially in critical care areas)
* Resistant TB
* Dengue fever
* Food-related outbreaks (such as E. coli)
* Malaria
* Norwalk
* Chicken pox
* Ebola
* Influenza
* Meningitis

Additional areas and groups to monitor include:
* Infections involving urinary catheters and other such indwelling devices
* Sharps or needle-stick injuries in staff
* Surgical-site infections (SSIs)

* Implanted device infections
* Infections within immunocompromised patient populations such as geriatric populations, neonatal populations, or patients on suppression therapy
* Infections in patients with chronic illnesses such as asthma, diabetes, heart disease, or HIV

More types of surveillance measures, their sources, and other information can be found at
http://www.qualitymeasures.ahrq.gov
Here's a brief look at some of them:
* Surgical infection prevention: percentage of patients who received prophylactic antibiotics consistent with current guidelines
* Surgical infection prevention: percentage of patients who received prophylactic antibiotics one hour prior to surgical incision
* Surgical infection prevention: percentage of patients whose prophylactic antibiotics were discontinued within 24 hours after surgery end time
* Influenza immunization: percentage of applicable patients receiving influenza immunizations (home-based primary care [HBPCI] cohort)
* Influenza immunization: percentage of applicable patients receiving influenza immunizations (spinal cord injury & disorders [SCI&D] cohort)
* Pneumonia: percentage of patients who were screened for pneumococcal vaccine status and were vaccinated prior to discharge, if indicated
* Pneumonia: median time from hospital arrival to administration of first antibiotic dose

Multiple Drug-Resistant Bacteria

Vancomycin Resistant Enterococcus (VRE)

Enterococci are bacteria that naturally live in the stomach which usually only cause infection when a person is sick. Vancomycin resistant enterococcus (VRE) is a bacterium that causes dangerous infections and can infect many different parts of the body.

Over the years, an increasing number of bacteria have mutated, becoming resistant to traditional antibiotics. VRE bacteria can't be killed by a powerful antibiotic medicine called vancomycin. Also, many other antibiotics used to fight infections can't kill VRE readily. Furthermore, VRE is extremely contagious, which makes it a major health concern for caregivers.

The reason that bacteria such as VRE become resistant to vancomycin is that healthcare workers have been using it before trying other antibiotics, even though vancomycin should usually be a "last resort" antibiotic treatment. VRE spreads from caregivers' hands and hospital equipment. It can live on gloves, instruments, countertops, and office surfaces.

Risk factors for VRE include:
* Long-term use of vancomycin or other antibiotics
* Illness of a life-long nature
* A weak immune system
* Use of intravenous (IV) drugs
* Liver or other organ transplant
* Dialysis treatments
* Proximity to a VRE carrier in the intensive care unit (ICU)
* Surgery in abdominal, pelvic, heart, brain, spinal cord, or other areas.
* Tube insertion, such as those for certain abdominal procedures, feeding tubes, and IV tubes.

The main symptoms of VRE include:
* The skin around the infected area becomes red and warm
* Energy level is low and the level of fatigue is high
* Fever
* Nausea and vomiting
* The site of infection is reddened and painful, usually with swelling and drainage.

To prevent patients from getting VRE:
* Never give a patient antibiotics for illnesses caused by a virus, since antibiotics cannot treat or cure viral infections. Not adhering to this is what allows bacteria to mutate, and antibiotics aren't necessary for viral conditions, as they generally go away with time.
* Patients being treated for bacterial infections with antibiotics should never stop taking them before the caregiver says so. Not adhering to this can also cause bacteria to become resistant to that particular antibiotic.
* Strictly follow hand hygiene procedures, particularly washing before touching food and after coughing, sneezing, a bowel movement, or visiting a patient who has VRE.

What is the treatment for VRE? Since VRE is resistant to many antibiotics, there currently are no definitive therapies for infections with VRE. Some of the attempts found to be useful in guiding drug therapy include susceptibility testing to all antimicrobial possibilities. This can include combination therapy involving the use of penicillins, vancomycin, and ampicillin, among others.

Another type of drug therapy belonging to a new class of drugs called the streptogramins is still under investigation. One such agent is Quinupristin-dalfopristin (Synercid®).

Without effective antibiotic interventions, caregivers can only treat VRE with fluid drainage, surgery, and precautions against contact.

What is MRSA (Methicillin-resistant *Staphylococcus aureus*)?

Staphylococcus Aureus is another bacterium that can sometimes cause dangerous infections. Usually, most Staphylococcus Aureus bacteria can be killed with antibiotics, such as methicillin, cephalosporins, nafcillin, and oxacillin. However, just as with VRE, this bacterium can mutate and become resistant to most antibiotics, including most penicillins and cephalosporins. Then it is called methicillin-resistant *Staphylococcus aureus* (MRSA).

There are a variety of ways in which people can become affected by MRSA infections:
* Without showing any symptoms of illness, it can be carried in the nose or on the skin (called MRSA colonization).
* Visible infections such as such as boils, wound infections, and pneumonia can also occur.

Like many other infections, direct contact from person to person is the primary method of MRSA spreading, particularly via the hands. To prevent the spread of MRSA, the usual, required hand hygiene should be adhered to after:
* The care of each patient
* Handling soiled dressings and clothing
* Wearing gloves.

Also, individuals in the healthcare environment should adhere to proper IC requirements for:
* Washing of hands before and after contact with every patient

* Avoidance of cross-contamination between clean and dirty linen
* Daily environmental cleaning
* Wearing gloves for all dressing changes
* Proper handling of infectious waste
* Observing isolation procedures
* Reporting illness including unusual skin rashes or boils to the nursing director prior to working with patients

No treatment is usually necessary for a person who carries MRSA, but doesn't exhibit any symptoms. The antibiotic vancomycin is not effective against MRSA when taken orally, but has been administered intravenously with varying levels of success. However, serious side effects can occur with vancomycin.

If the MRSA causes a serious infection, other antibiotics can be used to treat it. If the MRSA is mild to moderately severe, trimethoprim-sulfamethoxazole or minocycline (Dynacin, Minocin, Vectrin) can be used to treat it (if susceptibility testing supports this). Most MRSA strains are currently susceptible to rifampin (Rifadin, Rimactane) and fusidic acid (not commercially available in the United States). However, because the risk of selecting resistant mutants during treatment is substantial, these agents should sometimes not be used alone.

A variety of new agents have been developed over the last few years that have shown to have in vitro activity against resistant gram-positive organisms such as MRSA. The streptogramin compound quinupristin-dalfopristin (Synercid) and the oxazolidinone linezolid (Zyvox) are two examples.

Currently under investigation, newer semisynthetic glycopeptides, lipopeptide daptomycin (Cidecin), and fluoroquinolones with enhanced in vitro activity have show to have some effectiveness against such gram-positive organisms as MRSA.

Personnel Issues

An oversight committee is made up of at least the following:
* An administrator
* A medical director,
* A quality management or performance improvement professional
* The person responsible for IC

This committee needs to have regular meetings to examine the collected IC data on:
* Infection occurrence and containment
* IC processes and procedures
* Process improvement opportunities

How can an organization be sure it involves all of its areas? To create, implement, and monitor the IC program, the organization can charge one of the following with creating, implementing, and monitoring the IC program:
* A multidisciplinary IC team
* A task force
* A formal committee

A multidisciplinary IC committee is extremely helpful in formulating and sustaining an effective IC program. A committee is required in some states by licensure law, regulations, or rules, but not specifically required by JCAHO. All related departments and all major clinical service areas should be broadly included in the multidisciplinary IC group, committee, or team. Some of these are:

* Central sterile processing
* Environmental services
* Equipment maintenance personnel
* Facilities management, including engineering and maintenance personnel
* Finance
* Housekeeping
* Human resources
* Information management (patient records and information technology [IT] staff)
* Laboratory
* Medical staff
* Nursing
* Patient safety
* Performance improvement (PI)
* Pharmacy
* Rehabilitation

Besides the fact that the meetings need to take place on a regular basis, the following should also be addressed:
* Active participation
* Action items
* Appropriate organization
* Deliverables and/ or next steps with time frames
* Responsible parties

Comprehensive, focused goals relating to infection, prevention, and control need to be developed as a beginning step. Some of the factors that can influence an organization's goals are:
* Characteristics of the patient population, such as demographics or geography
* Type of care, treatment, and services provided
* Locally adopted clinical pathways or practice guidelines
* Current local, state, and federal laws

* Results of past studies, audits, or clinical findings
* Information from the Centers for Disease Control and Prevention (CDC) and other public health agencies on emerging pathogens and bioterrorist events

When the team constructs the plan, they should make sure that they cover infection prevention and control issues relating to:
* Patients
* Licensed independent practitioners (LIPs)
* Staff
* Volunteers
* Students
* Trainees
* Visitors

It's important for the team to ensure that these written policies and procedures:
* Are clear
* Outline the departments included in the plan
* Are short and useful

How can an organization make sure that its IC program addresses all the issues?
* By having a designated individual with IC experience take the lead in constructing the program
* By making sure that person obtains feedback during the creation process from other appropriate areas of the organization, such as clinical or pharmacy staff.
* By sharing IC plans with the organization's quality improvement committee, so as to get feedback and suggestions for improvement.

The IC practitioner is responsible for leading the organization in the areas of surveillance, outbreak control, and the use of isolation and other precautions.

In the surveillance area, the IC professional (ICP) needs to:
* Collect data on individual cases
* Figure out whether a nosocomial (of hospital origin) infection is present
* Assess and report the data to the oversight committee
* Making sure that regular rounds of the facility to evaluate IC practices are conducted

In the area of outbreak control, the ICP needs to:
* First figure out whether an outbreak has happened
* Use data collected in surveillance to analyze the situation
* Respond swiftly via isolation, mass vaccination, etc.

With the use of isolation and other precautions, the ICP will:
* Work with all staff to help prevent cross-infections
* Supervise the use of barrier methods long familiar to hospitals
* Get expertise from the Environment of Care (EC) staff on ventilation and water systems design and maintenance.

Policies and procedures for IC need to include details for the following hospital departments and services:
* Dietary
* Laundry
* Rehabilitation
* Respiratory
* Medication administration services
* Hand hygiene practices (key area)
* Multi-dose medication vial protocols (key area)

All staff needs to be educated in basic IC principles, as well as how to recognize early problem and symptom in both residents and themselves. Specifically, each staff member should be trained on:
* Disease transmission
* Hand hygiene—why, when, and how
* Standard precautions
* Basic hygiene
* Early recognition of infection problems or symptoms
* Proper use and disposal of sharps
* Proper use of new safety devices
* Handling of regulated medical waste

There are some measures that a hospital or other healthcare organization can take to prevent and control the spread of HAIs. Some of them include:
* Not eating or drinking occurs when care is delivered or where care recipients are seen
* Making certain that hand washing areas are equipped with paper towels, trash cans, and appropriate soap
* Mandating that good housekeeping is performed regularly for dust and odor control
* Only allowing approved disinfectants to be present on the unit and that they are used appropriately
* Ensuring that face shields, goggles, and personal protective equipment (PPE) are available and used during procedures and in cleaning
* Keeping sharps containers secured at all times and emptied when three-quarters full
* Making sure that linen bags are free of holes or tears and are emptied when two-thirds full
* Requiring that all items, especially instruments, are transported through the facility in a closed cart or biohazard bag

* Keeping all high-level disinfection and sterilization logs maintained appropriately.
* For restrooms, being aware of the added challenges for toilets, sinks, faucets, flushing handles, paper towel dispensers, and doors. For example, if sinks are too shallow, they might harbor bacteria in the drain.

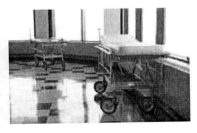

Some other hospital areas that demand special scrutiny are preoperative and recovery rooms, and nurses' stations.
Preoperative and recovery room considerations include:

* IV stands
* Monitoring equipment
* Beds
* Gurneys

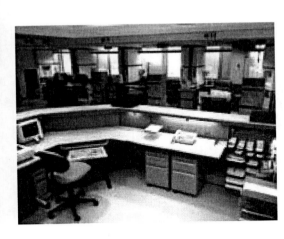

Nurses' station concerns include:
* Computers
* Keyboards
* Mouse
* Monitor
* Charts
* Writing instruments
* Counters
* Desk surfaces

In both of these areas, protective coverings need to be removed and replaced as soon as possible:
* When they become overtly contaminated
* At the end of a work shift if they might have been contaminated during the shift
Examples of this include coverings such as plastic wrap or aluminum foil.

Also critical for these areas is the scrutiny of reusable containers, which need to be inspected and decontaminated:
* On a regularly scheduled basis
* Immediately or as soon as feasible when visibly contaminated
Bins, pails, and cans, are examples of these.

These areas further demand that special attention be paid to broken glassware which, when broken, should:
* Only be picked up with mechanical means, such as a brush and dustpan or tongs. Not be touched with bare hands

The organization should have a resident health program that deals with:
* Immunizations (possibly missing by many residents)
* Personal hygiene
* Testing for latent TB infection on admission

There should also be an employee health program, since their health is paramount and needs to be assessed both:
* Initially upon hiring
* On an ongoing basis

Also, there should be an antibiotic review to help the facility construct a strategy for control of antibiotic-resistant organisms throughout the organization.

Finally, the organization needs to have disease-reporting protocols to:
* Check state health departments for reportable diseases
* Have a system in place for reporting them

Detailed Prevention Procedures

A common theme of this course is that the best way to halt the spread of infection is through comprehensive hand hygiene. This seems to be a major challenge for many health care organizations, despite the fact that cleaning hands is not a difficult act.

Some of the problems are that staff don't clean their hands as well as they should because they:
 * Are too busy
* Are too distracted
* Don't respect the importance of stringent hand hygiene

But the simple truth is that good hand hygiene is:
* A chief measure in breaking the chain of infection
* A major part of any effective IC program
* A requirement of the National Patient Safety Goals and Standards.
* Must be implemented throughout the organization per CDC guidelines

There are some definite ways in which healthcare organizations can better their staff's execution of correct hand hygiene throughout the organization. Staff members must be educated, since some workers don't realize what job activities can cause hand contamination. Some things are obvious to workers, such as washing hands after dressing an open wound. But some may be less obvious, like assisting a Caesarean patient in standing up and walking. This, too, requires subsequent hand washing.

Another issue is that a lot of healthcare professionals don't see the cause-and-effect connection between good hand hygiene and infection prevention, since there's a delay between inadequate hand cleaning and the appearance of an infection.

Organizations need to give workers information on these matters during staff in-services, on patient and break room wall posters, or via in-house e-bulletins and newsletters. This information should cover:
* The importance of proper hand hygiene
* How to engage in it at appropriate times
* Real statistics that illustrate the detriments of noncompliance
This education has to go even further, since hand hygiene sometimes needs to be accomplished with different cleansing agents and techniques, for example:
* Hand washing
* Hand rubs

Workers should wash hands with soap and water when they are:
* Visibly dirty or contaminated with organic material
* Visibly soiled with blood or other body fluids

For the routine decontamination of hands that aren't visibly soiled, staff can use soap and water or an alcohol-based hand rub.

Healthcare facilities should create and foster an organization-wide culture that promotes hygiene. In fact, the unacceptability of noncompliance should be a normal mindset for the entire staff. As an illustration of this, even the chief of surgery should be told not to enter an operating room (OR) and touch a patient without first doing a pre-operative hand prep.

The culture should make every worker comfortable in saying, "I'm sorry, but, unfortunately, you have to leave and do your hand prep before coming back in."

If any member of the staff isn't comfortable with bringing this to any other person's attention, no matter what their level of authority, then the organization hasn't created the proper hand-hygiene culture. Studies show that good leadership does encourage workers to remind them, and this increases the likelihood that workers will follow the protocols.

This changing of mindsets can take some time, due to the slow nature of behavioral changes which can sometimes be:
* Hard to initiate
* Slow to take hold
* In need of regular reminders of correct behavior

Here are some ways in which an organization can track changes in culture, as well as to look for areas needing improvement:
* Monitor general hand-hygiene adherence
* Give personnel feedback about their performance
* As a specific example, continually check the volume of alcohol-based hand rub used per 1,000 patient days
* Conduct observational studies of hand-washing practices and hand-rub use

The organization needs to make hand hygiene easy and convenient for workers. If noncompliance is a result of high volume, sometimes a helpful intervention is to provide alcohol-based hand rubs so as to:
* Make hygiene procedures quicker

* Increase effectiveness
* Enhance overall hand-hygiene compliance

Some of the locations in which these hand rubs can be made readily available include:
* Inside the entrance to the patient's room
* At the patient's bedside
* In other convenient locations
* In individual pocket-sized containers to be carried by care givers

It is imperative that the hand hygiene rules have the support of clinical leaders, since other caregivers follow their lead. When general personnel see clinical leaders regularly performing hand washing or hand antisepsis, it encourages them to:
* Follow their example
* Feel more comfortable in speaking up when they see others neglecting the rules

This leadership includes:
* Doctors
* Nurses
* Informal leaders

Education needs to be provided to patients and their families about hand washing, and everyone needs to be able to question the healthcare providers about whether their hands have been washed.

A helpful reminder from a patient of this crucial infection-control strategy can go a long way for busy and hectic staff members. Example: All staff can wear buttons that read, "Ask me if I've washed my hands."

One important fact is that some staff members mistakenly rely solely on gloves. This isn't a valid strategy, despite the fact that gloves do have a major role in preventing infection spreads. But gloves have their limitations because:
* They might have tiny perforations that allow pathogens to reach the skin
* Staff members may forget to remove gloves after touching a patient and before entering another area
* Bacteria can be spread from one part of the body to another if staff do not replace soiled gloves between tasks
* Touching surfaces such as door handles or telephones with used gloves can also spread bacteria

Therefore, staff members need to:
* Remove gloves after use
* Be educated on when gloves are appropriate
* Carry out hand washing and hand antisepsis (regardless of glove use) before and after each patient contact

Here's how to use an alcohol-based hand rub to decontaminate hands:
1) Base how much of the product to use on the manufacturer's recommendations
2) Apply product to palm of one hand
3) Rub hands together
4) Cover all surfaces of hands and fingers
5) Continue until hands are dry.

And here is how hands should be washed when using soap and water:
1) Wet hands with water (don't use hot water because repeated exposure to hot water can increase the risk of dermatitis)
2) Apply an amount of product recommended by the manufacturer to hands. (Liquid, bar, leaflet, or powdered forms

of plain soap are acceptable when washing hands with a non-antimicrobial soap and water. When bar soap is used, soap racks that facilitate drainage and small bars of soap should be used.)

3) Rub hands together vigorously for at least 15 seconds
4) Cover all surfaces of the hands and fingers
5) Rinse hands with water
6) Dry thoroughly with a disposable towel.
7) Make to sure use a towel to turn off the faucet.

In healthcare settings, the use of multiple-use cloth towels of the hanging or roll type is not suggested.

This is how to perform surgical hand antisepsis:

1) Remove rings, watches, and bracelets before beginning the surgical hand scrub.
2) Remove debris from underneath fingernails using a nail cleaner under running water.
3) Before putting on sterile gloves for surgical procedures, either an antimicrobial soap or an alcohol-based hand rub should be used.
4) If using an antimicrobial soap, scrub hands and forearms for 2 to 6 minutes or what the product's manufacturer recommends. It's not necessary to scrub for longer periods of time (e.g., 10 minutes).
5) If using an alcohol-based surgical hand-scrub product, follow the manufacturer's instructions. Before applying the alcohol solution, pre-wash hands and forearms with a non-antimicrobial soap and dry hands and forearms completely.
6) Allow hands and forearms to dry thoroughly before putting on sterile gloves.

Many factors go into the selection of effective hand-hygiene agents. The products should be both efficacious and have a low potential for irritancy, especially if they'll be used many times during a shift.

Whether the products are used for hand antisepsis before and after patient care in clinical areas, or used for surgical hand antisepsis by surgical personnel, these suggestions should be followed.

The cost of products should be secondary to making sure employees will accept them. So other factors take priority, such as the feel, fragrance, and skin tolerance, and workers should be asked for their input and preferences. This will better ensure that the employees will follow the procedures with the necessary rigor.

It's important to get manufacturer information about known interactions of their hand-cleaning products with:
* Non-antimicrobial soaps
* Antimicrobial soaps
* Alcohol-based hand rubs
* Skin care products
* Types of gloves used in the institution

To ensure that dispensers operate correctly and deliver a proper amount of product, evaluate the dispenser systems of several product manufacturers or distributors prior to making purchasing decisions. Never "top off" dispensers by adding soap to a partially empty soap dispenser, since bacterial contamination of soap can result.

To mitigate the risks of irritant contact dermatitis associated with hand antisepsis or handwashing, healthcare employees should be supplied with hand lotions or creams.

Again, information should be obtained from the product manufacturers regarding interactions between the persistent effects of antimicrobial soaps being used at the facility and their hand lotions, creams, or alcohol-based hand antiseptics.

There are some general considerations to follow in the interest of good IC hand hygiene:
* When having direct contact with patients at high risk (for example, those in ICUs or ORs), don't wear artificial fingernails or extenders .
* Never let natural nails tips get more than 1/4-inch long.
* When having contact with blood or other potentially infectious materials, mucous membranes, and non-intact skin, always don gloves first.
* After caring for a patient, make sure to remove gloves.
* Never wear the same pair of gloves for the care of more than one patient.
* Don't wash gloves between uses with different patients.
* If moving from a contaminated body site to a clean body site, change gloves during patient care.
* Wearing rings in health care settings seems to be acceptable, since no recommendations have been established.

Although some of these items were discussed earlier, the following is a checklist of important items for management to monitor throughout the facility on a continual basis:
* Hand hygiene facilities need to be adequate in number and used.
* The placement of hand hygiene facilities needs to encourage their use.
* Dispensers for alcohol-based hand rubs need to be placed at or near the entrances to appropriate patient and other rooms, as well as inside patient rooms.

* The placement of hand rub dispensers needs to conform to applicable local and federal codes.
* Hand rub dispensers need to be properly maintained.
* Staff needs to know correct hand hygiene techniques.
* Staff needs to understand the term "standard precautions."
* Staff needs to know how to use personal protective equipment, including utility gloves (for EC staff)
* The organization culture needs to encourage any staff member to remind another to practice hand hygiene if non-adherence is observed.

The risks of needle sticks and other sharps injuries exist for more than just clinical staff. Such hazards also exist for EC (Environment of Care) employees, such as:
* Housekeepers
* Sanitation workers
* Laundry workers

The Occupational Safety and Health Administration (OSHA) mandates that healthcare organizations train personnel to use needle safety devices to battle the threat of bloodborne infection. However, too many risky behaviors still exist, such as not manually recapping and not properly disposing of needles and sharps.

This indicates that there is a need for more of the current sharps safety products, such as:
* Needleless IV delivery systems
* Needles that retract into a syringe or vacuum tube holder
* Hinged or sliding shields attached to phlebotomy needles
* Winged-steel needles
* Blood gas needles

But unless healthcare personnel throughout the organization are trained on the correct and consistent use of these new devices, they aren't worth very much.

Workers also need to be taught to alert patients to the hazards of needles and sharps exposure.

According to the OSHA Bloodborne Pathogens Standard's minimum design performance elements for sharps disposal, containers should be:
* Closable,
* Puncture-resistant
* Leak proof on the sides and bottom
* Labeled or color-coded in accordance with the standard

Unused, discarded sharps are considered to be regulated medical waste.

For an organization to determine which of the countless available containers it should choose, it needs to do an assessment of its own risks, including:
* Workplace hazards (biological, physical, chemical, and radiological hazard containment needs)
* Size and type of sharps to be disposed of
* Volume of sharps to be disposed of at each point of use
* Frequency of sharps disposal container emptying and mounting bracket servicing by maintenance staff

Performance Criteria for Sharps Disposal Containers

In the area of functionality, containers need to stay in working order throughout the full period of their usage. They also need to be:

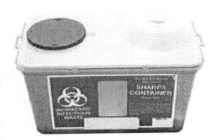

* Disposable
* Closable
* Leak resistant on their sides and bottoms
* Puncture resistant until final disposal
* Sufficient in number, with proper volume and safe access to the disposal opening.

Some of the functional criteria include:
* Barrier material performance
* Closure mechanisms
* Stability
* Size and shape
* Mounting brackets.
The containers should be capable of being reached by all employees who use, maintain, or dispose of sharp devices. They also need to be conveniently placed and portable, if appropriate, within the workplace. Some criteria of accessibility include:
* Disposal opening
* Access mechanism
* Handles
* General location and placement
* Installation height

The containers need to be seen plainly by the workers who will be using them. Employees also need to be able to see proper warning labels and color coding, as well as how full that container is. Some of the criteria for visibility include:
* The presence of hazard warning labels in accord with OSHA's bloodborne pathogens standard, which states, "These labels shall be fluorescent orange or orange-red or predominantly so, with lettering or symbols in a contrasting color, and display the

biohazard symbol and the word Biohazard." Red bags or containers may be substituted for labels.

* Lighting conditions need to be:
-- Adequate to display the container's fill status
-- Free from safety features or security measures that distort recognition of container, opening or access, warning labels, or fill status.

The design of containers should allow for convenient use by the worker and the facility. Containers also should be environmentally sound (e.g., made of recycled materials and free of heavy metals). Further, the design needs to make it easy to assemble, operate, and store the containers.

Here are some criteria related to accommodation:
* Worker training requirements
* Flexibility in design
* One-handed disposal
* Minimal sharp surfaces or cross-infection hazards
* Simple mounting used only for the specified container

Training needs to be implemented regarding:
* Assembly instructions
* Safety considerations
* Maintenance criteria for reusable containers
* Optimum storage conditions
* Warranty information
* Decontamination recommendations
* Container retirement considerations
* Bilingual or multilingual material where needed
* Sharps disposal container disposal considerations
* Information for periodic in-service training if required

When trying to control infections in hospital, behavioral health, and long-term care organizations, one of the most important functions to monitor is the handling of food. Besides adhering to local and federal agency regulations, the following procedures should be followed:

* Food should be properly stored, paying strict attention to temperature and security.
* Both food and nonfood items need to be correctly labeled.
* No food should be obtained from any source that doesn't process food under quality and sanitation controls that are regulated.
* The processes of making, storing, and dispensing ice need to follow procedures that will prevent contamination.
* Food items that can be accessed by both patients and their families (including food from the home) need to be stored properly.
* When cutting meat, fish, poultry, raw fruits and vegetables (as well as cooked foods), only sanitized cutting boards should be used, and they should be either nonabsorbent or used separately.
* Following each use, work surfaces need to be cleaned.
* To stop moisture, condensation, and the growth of mold, there must be proper control of lighting, ventilation, and humidity.

Besides the recommendations for the food items, the handlers (workers) should follow proper employee health requirements and procedures, such as:

* Physical examinations should be required on a routine basis
* Workers with open, infected wounds shouldn't be allowed to prepare food.
* Specific hand-washing methods need to be employed by workers with any kind of wound.
* Workers need to be compelled to wear clean, washable clothing, along with hair caps or nets.

* Workers should not be allowed to eat, drink, or smoke in areas designated for the preparation of food.
* The washing of dishes and utensils needs to have the correct amount of space and to follow the proper safety techniques.
* China, glassware, plastic ware, utensils, and disposables need to be done correctly
* Traffic needs to be controlled in food-service areas
* The holding, transfer, and disposal of garbage need to be conducted properly.
* Workers in the laundry area should not be allowed to eat, drink, smoke, chew gum, or apply cosmetics or makeup.
* All regular safeguards for the handling of soiled linens need to be followed.
* Also, when handling linens, workers need to use proper barriers such as reusable (rubber) gloves and aprons or gowns that prevent soak-through. Therefore, these items and the appropriate training on their use must be provided to workers.
* The soiled room must be equipped with a hygienic sink, paper towels, and soap dispensers as part of its required facilities for hand washing,
* Workers who handle soiled linens need to be in-serviced on methods for picking up sharps from linens or floors safely.
* Soiled linen should be handled as little as possible and with the least amount of agitation so that gross microbial contamination of the air and surfaces and of persons handling the linen will be avoided.
* Every soiled linen item should be placed in containers at the location where it was used before transporting, not sorted or rinsed at that location. IC procedures don't require that linen hampers have covers.
* In cases were laundry chutes are employed, all soiled linen needs to be bagged at the location where it was used before transporting, not sorted or rinsed at that location.

* If linen is heavily contaminated with blood or other body fluids, it should be bagged and carried in a way that stops it from leaking during transport.
* Personnel who sort soiled linen should be required to wear gloves and other protective garb as appropriate.

OSHA (The Occupational Safety and Health Administration) offers additional recommendations to safeguard workers from exposure to blood and other potentially infectious materials that could contaminate linens because of improper handling and labeling. Some of these are:
* When transporting contaminated laundry, it needs to be put in red bags and containers, or labeled with the biohazard symbol.
* Alternative labeling or color-coding is okay if it allows all workers to recognize the containers as requiring compliance with standard precautions. This is only the case in a facility that uses standard precautions in the handling of all soiled laundry.
* Red bags or bags marked with the biohazard symbol must be used in facilities that don't use standard precautions for all laundry.
* To avoid punctures from improperly discarded syringes, contaminated laundry bags shouldn't be squeezed or held too close to the body during transport.

Hierarchy of Decontamination

There are 4 kinds of cleaning in what has become known as the "hierarchy of decontamination of equipment and supplies." They are:
* Cleaning
* Decontaminating
* Disinfecting
* Sterilizing

In addition to health care worker hands, pathogens can find harbor in handled items. Some of these include improperly cleaned equipment, like:
* Surgical instruments
* IV poles
* Endoscopes

Also, capable of transmitting infections between patients and staff members (or from one to the other) are supplies, such as:
* Bed sheets
* Patient gowns
* Eating utensils

Workers who maintain and repair equipment and those who handle laundry are just as at-risk for exposure as direct care staff can be.

The following procedures and policies need to be instituted so as to assure the proper cleaning of equipment and supplies:
* Equipment and supplies that require cleaning, in contrast with those that are disposable.
* The timing for mandatory cleaning (when)
* The frequency of cleaning (how often)
* The method of cleaning (technique)

The organization's policies need to be developed with the collaboration of various departments, including:
* Nursing
* IC professionals
* Housekeeping
* Food service
* Biomedical staff

In addition to direct care staff, the people who repair and maintain equipment and clean soiled laundry need to be protected from contamination, and hence should be involved in making policies, even if the organization doesn't have on-site biomedical or laundry staff.

Prior to and following each patient use, equipment needs to be cleaned thoroughly. When equipment is used from one department to another, it should also be cleaned. Before a piece of equipment gets to an equipment maintenance department, it should be properly decontaminated. Then, before returning to the direct care environment, it should be decontaminated again.

As mentioned earlier, four types of cleaning are used to rid equipment of dirt and pathogens. Which one to use in a given situation is determined by the type of equipment and its intended use.

The first method is simply called "cleaning," and its purpose is to get rid of all visible dust, soil, and any other visible material that microorganisms might find favorable for continued life and growth. Scrubbing with hot water and detergent can usually achieve this.

The second method is called "decontamination," and is employed to remove disease-producing organisms. This makes the equipment safe to handle.

The third method is called "disinfection," and is used to kill most disease-producing organisms, although not all microbial forms can be removed with this process. Actually, there are three levels of disinfection:

* High level: All organisms except high levels of bacterial spores are killed with an FDA-approved germicide (FDA=Food and Drug Administration).
* Intermediate level: Mycobacteria, most viruses, and bacteria are killed with a chemical germicide registered as a tuberculocide by the Environmental Protection Agency (EPA).
* Low level: Some viruses and bacteria are killed using a chemical germicide registered as a hospital disinfectant by the EPA.

The fourth method of cleaning is called "sterilization," and causes all types of microbial life to die. This includes:
* Bacteria
* Viruses
* Spores
* Fungi
What actually is sterilization? Using a procedure, either physical or chemical, to kill all microbial life (highly resistant bacterial endospores included).

Some of the ways in which hospitals sterilize equipment and supplies include:
* Steam autoclaving
* Ethylene oxide gas
* Dry heat

Many new chemical germicides have been found effective in allowing hospitals to reprocess expensive reusable equipment, such as endoscopes and other heat-sensitive medical devices.

Different sterilization methods have both their advantages and disadvantages. Examples:
* Liquid sterilizers only work when the device is able to be immersed in the fluid

* Oxidative formulations can do damage to rubber and plastics. Peracetic acid and hydrogen peroxide are not exempt.

E.H. Spaulding developed a classification system over 30 years ago for figuring out the best equipment cleaning methods. When healthcare organizations need to classify their equipment for decontamination, looking at Spaulding's system is a good place to begin. There are three classes of patient care items, based, not on the potential contamination level, but on the intended use of the device instead.
* Critical
* Semi critical
* Non-critical

To illustrate, the category of "non-critical" means that the degree of infection injury to workers and patients isn't critical, not that the items can't contain contaminants.

The following is a breakdown of how each category should be cleaned:
Critical items need to be sterilized. These can include:
* Items used to enter or contact sterile tissues
* Instruments entering a surgical incision
* Implants, and needles placed into the vascular system.

Semi-critical items need high-level disinfection. Items under this category are:
* Items that come into contact with non-intact skin or mucous membranes
* Respiratory therapy equipment
* Anesthesia equipment
* Flexible endoscopes

Non-critical items need basic cleaning and low-level decontamination. In this class are:
* Items that touch only intact skin
* Crutches
* Blood pressure cuffs

Different methods used to sterilize items have different advantages and disadvantages. Some of the main techniques as well as their positive and negative aspects in regards to an infection control program follow.

One of the advantages of steam sterilization is that in healthcare organizations, it's the most prevalent sterilization process. Another is that it's safe for workers in environmental and healthcare departments. On the negative side, however, this method of sterilization can face jeopardy from:
* Trapped air
* Grossly wet materials
* Decreased steam quality

Dry heat sterilization has different advantages, since it:
* Results in low corrosiveness
* Can penetrate deep into the material
* Is safe for the environment
* Doesn't require aeration
Negative aspects of dry heat sterilization include:
* The necessity for long sterilization time
* Conflicting requirements of different countries regarding temperature and cycle time
* Heat-labile component susceptibility to damage

The technique of sterilizing with 100% Ethylene oxide (ETO) has other advantages. Major positives include the fact that this process:

* Can penetrate packaging materials and lots of plastics
* Is compatible with most medical materials
* Is easy to operate and monitor
Here are some downsides to this technique:
* Aeration time is necessary
* The sterilization chamber is small
* The ETO substance is flammable, toxic, and a probable carcinogen
* Flammable liquid storage cabinets have to be used to store ETO cartridges

The hydrogen peroxide plasmasterilization process of sterilization has its own advantages, including the facts that it:
* Has a low process temperature
* Doesn't require aeration
* Is safe for healthcare and environmental workers
• Doesn't have toxic residuals
• Is easy to operate, install, and monitor
Disadvantages with this method include the problems incurred because it:
* Can't process cellulose, linens, and liquids
* Requires a small sterilization chamber
* Can't process medical devices with long or narrow lumen
* Needs synthetic packaging

Sterilization with formaldehyde has the advantages of being:
* Not explosive or flammable
* Compatible with most medical materials
Some of the negative aspects of formaldehyde sterilization are the facts that this process:
* Has the potential for residual formaldehyde on the surface
* Has a toxic and allergenic agent (formaldehyde)
* Needs a long sterilization time

* Requires a long processing time because, after sterilization, the formaldehyde has to be removed

CDC (The Centers for Disease Control and Prevention) has established suggestions for preventing infections such as nosocomial pneumonia. One method involves using sterile water to rinse nebulization devices and other semicritical respiratory-care equipment after they are cleaned and disinfected.

Another procedure can be used if the availability of sterile water is an issue. Filtered or tap water can be used for a preliminary washing step, then the equipment can be rinsed with isopropyl alcohol. Finally, forced air or a drying cabinet can be used to dry the item. Other important points:
* All water designated for filling nebulization device reservoirs MUST be sterile.
* The organization MUST provide comprehensive and intensive training for all staff members assigned to reprocessing equipment and supplies, no matter what processes, agents, and equipment will be used.
* Employees need to ask the organization's IC professional any questions on the proper cleaning, disinfection, or sterilization of any given device. The IC professional needs to consult with the device's manufacturer if uncertain of that proper procedure.

To prevent recontamination following the sterilization process, equipment and utensils need to be wrapped or packaged. The following steps can help achieve success with these procedures:
* To help protect instruments, compartmentalize containers
* For the best sterile barrier, be certain that the lip of the container fits securely
* Make sure that the size of the container is appropriate for the task

* Conduct daily tests to be certain that the package sealer is providing a uniform seal and adequate purchase. Never neglect to test the sealer after an item is sealed... and after it is sterilized, as well.
* Be certain that peel pouches are of a large enough size to allow the package to expand and contract without damaging either the instrument or the packaging.
* Make certain that no packaging is without an indicator or label.
* Be sure to always write on or apply a label to the plastic or polypropylene side of a peel pack.
* Constantly see to it that ink isn't bleeding through and creating a portal for bacteria.
* Prior to applying a dust cover, make sure that products are first cooled down.
* Make sure that only one- or two-layered sterilization trays are used, since using more can cause the sterilization process to be compromised.

Also, be certain that all wrapping materials used:
* Have enough durability to withstand punctures and tears
* Don't generate nonviable particles
* Are impervious to bacteria
* Are sealable prior to sterilization
* Are flexible enough to allow swift wrapping and unwrapping

Some particular recommendations for wrapping materials:
* Muslin needs to have a thread count of at least 140 threads per square inch
* At least two thicknesses of paper or non-woven fabric are necessary for other suitable materials, which include Kraft paper, paper or plastic peel-down packages, and non-woven wraps.

For cleaning laundry, a method of separating dirty linen and scrubs from clean linen must be developed by every organization. According to the CDC items should be laundered for a minimum of 25 minutes in at least 160-degree water or with chlorine bleach to remove pathogens from soiled laundry such as bed sheets and gowns.

Workers handling laundry need to wash their hands after touching contaminated laundry, and eating, drinking, or smoking in the workplace must be prohibited. To prevent clean linen and supplies from becoming contaminated by mopping of the floors, they should be stored at least 6 inches off the floor.

Splash and splatter from mopping activities can contaminate the exterior surface of linens and pose an infection risk to staff who handle them, even when enclosed in plastic wrap. Even when linens are enclosed in plastic wrap, splash and splatter from mopping activities can contaminate the exterior surface and pose an infection risk to laundry workers.

Organizations need to cover the ways that facility areas will be cleaned and disinfected, just as it must address this for equipment and supplies. Infection-causing microorganisms can breed in cooling towers, air ventilation systems, drains, ice machines, carpeting and flooring, elevator shafts, and garbage disposal areas. Policies and procedures should address these areas as well as equipment.

When designing policies and procedures for equipment cleaning, organizations must make sure that such policies and procedures apply to all equipment within the organization, including the equipment not owned by the organization, such as demonstration, substitute, loaner or rental units.

Because such equipment moves from organization to organization and is exposed to an unknown variety of potentially infectious agents, safe practices must include appropriate cleaning of equipment before it enters and before it exits the organization.

Organization staff needs to be trained and educated on the IC policies once the IC staff develops them. This includes biomedical personnel and nurses. Staff needs to be reminded by their organizations about:
* Which equipment should be cleaned
* What cleaning method should be used
* How often cleaning should occur
* Making sure that labels are on the equipment that are noticeable and easy to read

Ensure that the appropriate staff is following all the procedures necessary to effectively clean equipment by using checklists. Another good tool to use is a logbook. One of these should always be available to record the performance of decontamination procedures. To be certain that correct cleaning procedures are being executed, these logbooks should be monitored regularly.

Emergency Management

Besides covering issues of healthcare-associated infections, a good IC program needs to create a foundation for coping with emergency IC events such as:
* New infection outbreaks, e.g., SARS (Severe Acute Respiratory Syndrome)
* Pandemics, e.g., influenza
* Bioterrorist attacks

When an organization has good plans for general disasters, its handling of an IC emergency will not be much different. But over a protracted length of time, this type of problem could overwhelm an organization's ability to continue providing quality care.

JCAHO requirements mandate that emergency management plans that mitigate, prepare for, respond to, and recover from emergencies be developed by healthcare organizations.

The first thing a healthcare organization's leaders need to do in getting prepared for emergencies is to become represented at all area wide emergency management meetings. The basis for the organization's planning for these types of events should be rooted in information about how the first-responder system works in all types of disasters and what federal agencies can and cannot do in varying time frames.

An illustration of this can be seen from the World Trade Center attacks of 9/11/01, where the first places of refuge for victims were nearby:
* Hospitals
* Assisted living apartments
* Nursing homes

Due to the intense amount of dust in the environment, simply providing light and fresh water became major issues.

Local, state, and federal representatives should be included in pondering "what-if" strategies, along with the healthcare organization's IC practitioner and other key staff.

A multitude of questions need to asked and answered when gearing up for an IC emergency. Some of the major ones are:

* What level of risk exists for the organization, and what response measures should be in place based on that risk? Illustration: there won't be the same bioterrorism preparedness plan in a home care agency in rural Iowa and an acute care hospital in Boston.
* How will the organization ascertain that an emergency is occurring?
* Who will decide that the emergency management plan should be activated?
IC professionals have to keep monitoring emerging reports from public health departments and the CDC, as well as stay on top of their internal surveillance data.
* What will the chain of command be during an emergency?
* How will effective communication be facilitated?
* What are the organization's available response options?
-- Shut down?
-- Limit services?
-- Restrict access?
-- Transfer patients off site?
-- Serve as the community's primary emergency facility?

In the case where the facility stays open, a different set of questions need to be answered regarding how it will manage the flow of people in and out of the building.
* How will infected patients be dealt with?
* How will isolation be effected, if necessary?
* How will the safety of patients isolated for IC be handled?
* How will the organization deal with a mass decontamination, if warranted?
* What circumstances will necessitate barrier precautions?
* How will staff be trained on the proper use of those precautions?
* Will both clinical and non-clinical staff be involved in the training?

* If warranted, how will a quarantine be executed?
* What support systems will be in place for staff?
* What are the community resources available?
* Who should be contacted and how should they be contacted?
* How will the IC emergency plan be integrated within the community?
* What community resources can work together?
* How will the plan be tested?

Periodic testing of an organization's emergency management plan is required by JCAHO. That's the only way to be certain that the IC component of the plan addresses all issues in the proper manner. Depending upon the infectious agent being battled, these questions will be answered in different ways.

When isolating a patient is warranted, this can be accomplished by:
* Putting the patient in a private room
* Making healthcare workers and visitors wear gloves, gowns, masks, or other protective gear.
* Limiting the patient's movement outside of the room
Visitors are often restricted to confine the spread of infection.

The emergency management plan needs to explain how the organization will isolate large numbers of patients and be sure that they get quick care that is documented and safe.

Procedures also need to be set up to manage the provisions of isolated patients, including supplies like linens, eating utensils, and clothing.

Prior to an influx of sick patients, healthcare organizations need to have an emergency supply source in place. A hospital can examine its current inventory of supplies, food, water, and bedding as a starting place.

A healthcare organization might initiate the following interventions during an IC emergency:
* Biological residue removal from first responders, victims, and families
* Isolation of the contamination
* Decontamination and/or treatment of patients
* Protection of staff, other patients, visitors, and the facility
* Reestablishment of normal service

Other issues that organizations must address include identifying:
* Where contaminated victims will be housed
* How and where they will be decontaminated, no matter what season it is
* How they will handle and store the variety of contaminated materials

The best place to decontaminate patients is outside the main facility, so that staff, equipment and other patients can be protected against becoming contaminated. During hot weather, other temporary structures can be employed to keep patients' privacy intact. Keeping the patients away from direct exposure to the elements is another reason to use these makeshift structures.

People can be washed in decontamination showers set up outside, so that they're cleaned prior to entering the facility. Areas designated for decontamination need to be downwind of clean areas in such cases.

It's not always possible to decontaminate patients outside. People often come into a health care facility already infected, unbeknownst to the organization.

Sometimes a part of the facility will need to be quarantined from the rest of the place. To prepare for this potentiality, organizations need to assess their facility's layout to ascertain whether:
* Their air-handling systems can be isolated or not, in the case where this may be necessary to prevent the spread of contaminants throughout the building
* Particular rooms, corridors, or entrances might be used to isolate or quarantine staff and patients

To cordon off hallways or other areas and separate contaminated areas from clean ones, the following equipment can be used if fire-rated:
* Plastic sheeting
* Duct tape
* Spring-loaded poles

When organizations are large, they may have great facilities for cleaning patients, such as decontamination rooms and showers. However, when organizations are smaller, they may have to concede that they're not able to deal with large-scale IC emergencies. These organizations should work within the community to combine resources in a manner that allows them to create strength in numbers.

How should a decontamination area be set up?
* One side should be deemed "dirty" and another side should be designated as "clean."
* Until they're decontaminated, all contaminated personnel, equipment, and victims should stay on the dirty side.

* The dirty side should consist of a triage station, treatment station, and decontamination area.
* Both ambulatory and non-ambulatory patients should be accommodated in the decontamination area.
* In order to minimize cross-contamination, patients should perform as much of the decontamination as possible.

Disposal of contaminated water is a major concern with mass decontamination:
* To prevent the tracking of contaminants into the clean areas, shower runoff needs to be controlled.
* Attaching a small tub to each decontamination shower area can create a temporary tank.
* Contaminated water can be pumped out to a larger holding area for further testing and decontamination.
* The water runoff shouldn't be allowed to go down the drain unless a disinfectant can neutralize the biological agent(s).

Of course, the decontamination of patients is only part of the concern. Equipment will need to be decontaminated as well. Some equipment may not pose any challenges for cleaning. However, some may be much harder to decontaminate, such as permanent negative air equipment.

An emergency management plan for IC must be in accord with the needs and resources of the community, regardless of the organizational size. All organizations and facilities have little choice other than to work with each other in:
* Identifying problems
* Isolating the issues
* Treating patients
* Returning to regular operations

Managers of organizations should only create an IC emergency plan in collaboration with representatives from all community agencies of potential impact. Every stakeholder needs to contribute to all response plans in a way that:
* Capitalizes on the unique strengths of the facilities and departments within the community
* Outlines the responsibilities of those organizations.

Some of the groups with which organizations should meet and coordinate response plans for emergencies include:
* All healthcare facilities in the region
    - Acute care facilities
    - Long-term care facilities
    - Ambulatory facilities
    - Behavioral healthcare centers
* Public service organizations
    - Police department
    - Fire department
    - Red Cross
    - Hazardous materials enforcement organizations
    - Emergency management department
* Public health departments in local and regional jurisdictions
* School, community centers, and other organizations in the area

What are some tips for creating an integrated response plan that addresses responsibilities for each organization as well as the communication strategies between them?
* Be certain that that the IC professional is an integral part of the planning, from the very beginning.
* Ensure that every organization and department has a designated representative to the overall emergency coordinating body.

* Make certain that each organization maintains its own emergency response plan.
* Make it clear to whom information about the emergency should be communicated, including public health organizations and a multi-organizational emergency management team.
* Develop multiple means of communication in case standard methods are unavailable, e.g., if phone or fax systems become disabled, organizations should have plans to use radio technology or wireless or Internet communication.
* Figure out temporary credentialing and privileging policies so that personnel can "float" between organizations if need be.
* Make it clear to whom volunteers are to report and delineate a clear line of supervision.
* Find out ways to transport patients to and from different facilities.

JCAHO standards dictate that certain types of healthcare organizations make arrangements to decontaminate victims of toxic radioactive, biological, and chemical poisoning if an IC emergency occurs. These include:
* Acute care hospitals
* Critical access hospitals
* Ambulatory care organizations
* Long-term care organizations
It's not mandated that all these organizations actually have their own decontamination facilities, only that they have arrangements to have access somewhere if needed. Acute care and critical access hospitals are advised, however, to have their own decontamination facilities.

When an IC event occurs due to a possible nuclear, biological, or chemical terrorism attack, patients' possessions may need to collected as evidence. However, due to the dangers associated with the spread of infection, the following are some recommended procedures:

* If ambulatory and non-ambulatory patients are able to undress without assistance, they should put their valuables (wallets, jewelry, cell phones, keys, and so on) in a clear, pre-labeled, plastic, resealable bag.
* Each person needs to place a form of picture identification in the bag so that it is visible from the outside.
* Patients' glasses, canes, hearing aids, and other ambulatory devices should stay with the patient.
* If the ambulatory and non-ambulatory patients can't undress without assistance, they should put their clothing in a pre-labeled paper bag.
* This bag should be placed in a large, clear, pre-labeled, plastic, resealable bag if the clothing is contaminated with a chemical agent that might pose a risk of secondary contamination.
* Patient and event information should be placed on the bag.

The following information needs to be on the label for each patient and event.
* Patient name
* Date of birth
* Medical record #
* Date
* Time
* How much and what kind of decontamination was on clothing prior to placing in bag (if known)
* Geographical site where contamination occurred.
    - This information is critical to the epidemiological surveillance of the event and causative agent and can include proximity to the release site, and location at the time of the event, etc.)

Healthcare workers need to adhere to the same bagging and labeling procedures outlined for patients if they are assisting patients who are unable to undress or bag their own clothing.

To help identify patients' belongings after an event, a Polaroid picture of the patient prior to clothing removal should be taken and attached to the labeled bag if this is at all possible.

The collection of clothing and valuables should be overseen by a hospital police officer or a city police officer. To maintain the chain of evidence, each bag should be stored separately so that they don't touch each other, if possible.

When the time comes for releasing possessions back to patients, local law enforcement and hospital policy should determine the procedure.

References and Resources

Meeting JCAHO's Infection Control Requirements, Joint Commission Resources, Senior editor: Ladan Cockshut-Miller, 2004
Infection Control Issues in the Environment of Care, Joint Commission Resources, Senior Editor: Kristine M. Miller, 2005
Hospital Accreditation Standards, Joint Commission Resources, 2004
Three Things You Can Do To Prevent Infection: A Speak Up (SM) safety initiative, Joint Commission Resources, PDF file
The UniversityOfHealthCare Bioterrorism series: Bioterrorism Anthrax, Bioterrorism Botulinum, Bioterrorism Hemorrhagic Viruses, Bioterrorism Plague, Bioterrorism Radiation, Bioterrorism Smallpox, Bioterrorism Tularemia, Bioterrorism Certificate Program, Bioterrorism Guidebook by Daniel Farb, M.D. and Bruce Gordon

Web sites:
Joint Commission on Accreditation of Healthcare Organizations
www.jcaho.org
American Hospital Association
www.hospitalconnect.com
Association for Professionals in Infection Control and Epidemiology, Inc.
www.apic.org
Centers for Disease Control and Prevention
www.cdc.gov
Infectious Diseases Society of America
www.idsociety.org
Society for Healthcare Epidemiology of America
www.shea-online.org

Printable Checklist for Infection Control

Some measures that a hospital or other healthcare organization can take to prevent and control the spread of HAIs include:

☐ Not eating or drinking occurs when care is delivered or where care recipients are seen

☐ Making certain that hand-washing areas are equipped with paper towels, trash cans, and appropriate soap

☐ Mandating that good housekeeping is performed regularly for dust and odor control

☐ Only allowing approved disinfectants to be present on the unit and that they are used appropriately

☐ Ensuring that face shields, goggles, and personal protective equipment (PPE) are available and used during procedures and in cleaning

☐ Keeping sharps containers secured at all times and emptied when three-quarters full

☐ Making sure that linen bags are free of holes or tears and are emptied when two-thirds full

☐ Requiring that all items, especially instruments, are transported through the facility in a closed cart or biohazard bag

☐ Keeping all high-level disinfection and sterilization logs maintained appropriately.

☐ For restrooms, being aware of the added challenges for toilets, sinks, faucets, flushing handles, paper towel dispensers, and doors.

For example, if sinks are too shallow, they might harbor bacteria in the drain. Some other hospital areas that demand special scrutiny are preoperative and recovery rooms, and nurses' stations.

Preoperative and recovery room considerations include:
☐ IV stands
☐ Monitoring equipment

- [ ] Beds
- [ ] Gurneys

Nurses' station concerns include:
- [ ] Computers
- [ ] Keyboards
- [ ] Mouse
- [ ] Monitor
- [ ] Charts
- [ ] Writing instruments
- [ ] Counters
- [ ] Desk surfaces

In both of these areas, protective coverings need to be removed and replaced as soon as possible:
- [ ] When they become overtly contaminated
- [ ] At the end of a work shift if they might have been contaminated during the shift

Examples of this include coverings such as plastic wrap or aluminum foil.

Also critical for these areas is the scrutiny of reusable containers, which need to be inspected and decontaminated:
- [ ] On a regularly scheduled basis
- [ ] Immediately or as soon as feasible when visibly contaminated

Bins, pails, and cans, are examples of these.

These areas further demand that special attention be paid to broken glassware which, when broken, should:
- [ ] Only be picked up with mechanical means, such as a brush and dustpan or tongs. Not be touched with bare hands

The organization should have a resident health program that deals with:

- ☐ Immunizations (possibly missing by lots of residents)
- ☐ Personal hygiene
- ☐ Testing for latent TB infection on admission

There should also be an employee health program, since their health is paramount and needs to be assessed both:

- ☐ Initially upon hiring
- ☐ On an ongoing basis

Also, there should be an antibiotic review to help the facility construct a strategy for control of antibiotic-resistant organisms throughout the organization.

Finally, the organization needs to have a disease reporting protocols to:

- ☐ Check state health departments for reportable diseases
- ☐ Have a system in place for reporting them.

Printable Hand Hygiene Checklist

The following is a checklist of important items for management to monitor throughout the facility on a continual basis:

- ☐ Hand hygiene facilities need to be adequate in number and used.
- ☐ The placement of hand hygiene facilities needs to encourage their use.
- ☐ Dispensers for alcohol-based hand rubs need to be placed at or near the entrances to appropriate patient and other rooms, as well as in patient rooms.

☐ The placement of hand rub dispensers needs to conform to applicable local and federal codes.
☐ Hand rub dispensers need to be properly maintained.
☐ Staff needs to know correct hand hygiene techniques.
☐ Staff needs to understand the term "standard precautions."
☐ Staff needs to know how to use personal protective equipment, including utility gloves (for EC staff)
☐ The organization culture needs to encourage any staff member to remind another to practice hand hygiene if non-adherence is observed?